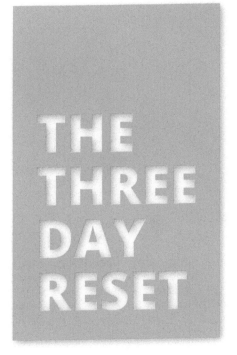

THE THREE DAY RESET

Heather Denniston DC CCWP

Author: Heather Denniston, DC CCWP - www.wellfitandfed.com

ISBN-13: 978-0-9897049-7-7

Cover and Layout Design: CreateHive

Editing: Red To Black Editing and Wordspark

Cover and Author Photo: Brandon Flint Photography

Printing: Gorham Printing

Printed in the United States of America

Contents

ACKNOWLEDGEMENTS

Like all authors, I am buoyed up by hands of many. Paula, from CreateHive, you made sure I had "dots" in all the right places. James Chestnut DC, your words from the stage sparked a deep passion for exceptional living. Kellyann Petrucci ND, although you were many steps ahead on the journey, you always had time to look back and say, "Come along!". My Caution girls, we've been glued at the hip for the last thirty years, and you had unrelenting belief in my small seeds of talent. My EPIC ladies, you provided prayers, encouragement and pressing in when I needed pressing. My "testing group" friends, you encouraged me by doing the program just because I said it was important to me. (Thanks for the panicky 8AM phone call about coffee, Mike. Yes, you can have a cup on the Reset.) And, of course, my sisters and mother who have always assumed I am capable of anything, even when I am not.

FOREWARD

As a kid, I was largely left to my own devices. My mother encouraged independence, my sisters were older, and my dad traveled. I found comfort in food. I quickly learned that food satiated more than my stomach. Loneliness, boredom, and restlessness all responded well to the ingestion of large amounts of calories. In addition to becoming a competitive overeater, I became addicted to sugar. It is no surprise that sugar triggers the same sensory areas of the brain as stimulant drugs. The ability to self-medicate with food is real. I was witness to food's power from the age of nine.

In the sixth grade, I attended a boarding school. Boarding school to a compulsive overeater is like sending a cocaine addict into a cozy crack den. With little supervision and access to a constant supply of food, things got worse. In college, my food behaviors spiraled and I became a nocturnal binger with no recollection of what or how much I had eaten in the middle of the night. My weight climbed to 235 pounds. I dieted, fell off the wagon, and dieted again, repeating the cycle dozens of times in desperation to lose the weight.

In my early twenties, I went off to chiropractic school, and suddenly, healthy people, passionate about exercise and optimal eating, surrounded me. I immersed myself in the study of nutrition and exercise and slowly started making changes. I started to feel more grounded and solidified in healthy interactions with food. I continued to implement and hone and refine.

With each new habit, my brain connection to nutrition slowly started to shift. The weight dropped and the bondage with food was dismantled. These transformations would mitigate my suffering with weight management and several autoimmune disorders over the next two decades. I finally felt I was healthy again and that I had a handle on what I should and should not be consuming.

The Three Day Reset is a culmination of my journey to understand the process by which we take in and use food as fuel and of how certain foods lead us directly to a fuller, healthier life experience. *The Three Day Reset's* intentional plan is designed to create the highest potential for success. I thank you for sharing this passion for exceptional health with me. I am forever grateful to my readers and participants in this program.

DEDICATION

To Moo. Thank you for saying,

"Live. Go do everything."

THE MISSION

To emotionally and physically step away from toxic, processed, and inflammatory foods, and to replenish our systems with whole, nutrient-rich alternatives.

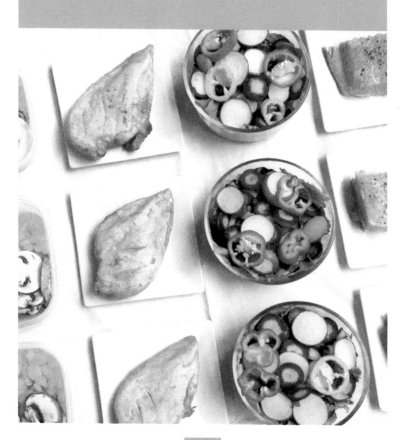

THE INTRO

After twenty years of studying and coaching patients on various nutrition protocols, I realized many people have similar frustrations when it comes to eating right. People's goals were consistent. They wanted "doable," clean, non-extreme methods to address moving toward healthier eating practices. With these goals in mind and with research across many sources and platforms, I developed *The Three Day Reset.*

The Three Day Reset is a gentle way to incorporate many of the best practices of the diverse programs I have found to be successful. The purpose of The *Three Day Reset* is to provide a framework through which we can start to build healthy food habits – habits that will spill over into our life outside "The Reset," habits that will result in a significant investment toward long-term abundant life experience, starting with nutrition. *The Three Day Reset* is not a diet.

It is a pause.
It is a respite for your innards.

The Three Day Reset gives your body a deeply needed break. The guidelines are simple, the shopping list straightforward. Upon completion, you will feel refreshed, renewed, and possibly, quite probably, you will be on your way to establishing lifelong healthy food habits.

THE WHATS

What is *The Three Day Reset?*

1. *The Three Day Reset* is a three day intentional food plan that will stimulate alkalization (establishing the best pH for digestion), cleaner processing of nutrients, and gentle detoxification of your body.

2. *The Three Day Reset* provides a break from all grains, dairy, sweeteners, legumes, nuts, seeds, eggs, processed foods, alcohol, soy, red meat, and pork. (Consider these foods your "**not allowed**" list.)

3. *The Three Day Reset* is a nutrition program that loads your body with vitamins, minerals, protein, and essential fats. It is not a crash diet (although you likely will lose weight); it is not a solution to counteract recent drinking or indulging.

4. *The Three Day Reset* is an opportunity for you to stop and evaluate how your body feels, free of the allergens, toxins, and chemicals common in our food.

5. *The Three Day Reset* allows us to enter into a practice of conscious eating, setting intention with every bite and taking time to ruminate on the fact that food is fuel, not friend. It is a focus on the fact that the cleaner the fuel, the better we run in all aspects of our existence.

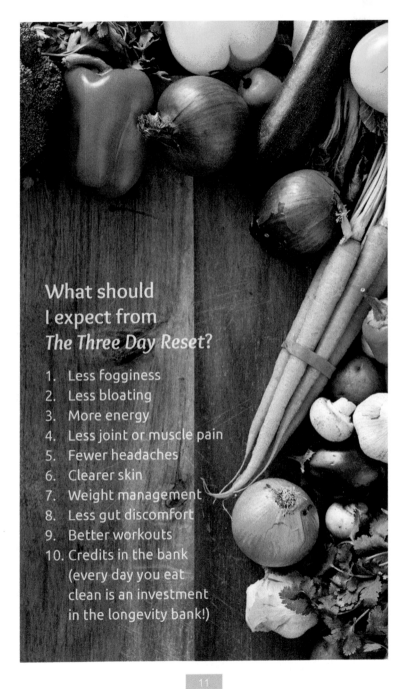

What should I expect from *The Three Day Reset?*

1. Less fogginess
2. Less bloating
3. More energy
4. Less joint or muscle pain
5. Fewer headaches
6. Clearer skin
7. Weight management
8. Less gut discomfort
9. Better workouts
10. Credits in the bank (every day you eat clean is an investment in the longevity bank!)

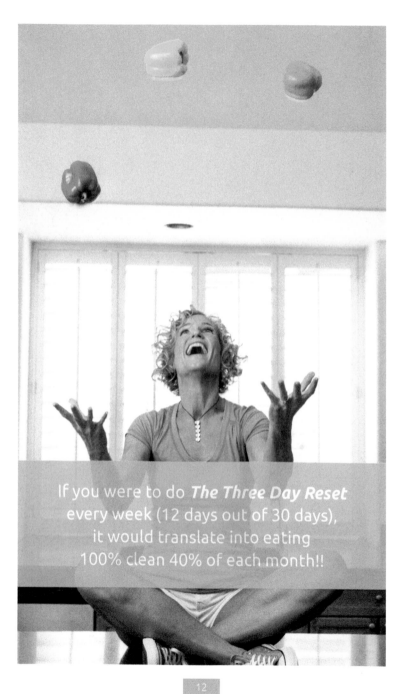

If you were to do *The Three Day Reset*
every week (12 days out of 30 days),
it would translate into eating
100% clean 40% of each month!!

THE INSTRUCTIONS

PICK

Choose three days you would like to do *The Three Day Reset*.

INFORM

Let your family and your other supporters know your plan so that they can prepare. (No friends calling last minute to go out for a drink or partners waving a big bowl of popcorn under your nose.)

SHOP

See shopping list details. Spend some time going through your cupboards and getting rid of things that are either going to be tempting or not in line with your goals.

PREP

Make sure that you have some prep time available the day before you start *The Three Day Reset*. I have my *Three Day Reset* prep down to 90 minutes. Allow 2 hours to 2.5 hours for your first couple of times. The more you accomplish during your prep time, the more successful you will be. You must set aside time to do this, or your journey will be much more difficult.

EXECUTE

Follow the "Execute" instructions. Remember that if you stick to the plan 100 percent, your results will be exceptional. Three days is doable for anyone and is a reasonable foray into healthy new practices in your life.

FEEL

Amazing!

REPEAT

At least one time a month (Preferably weekly!)

THE 40 PERCENT

I was a patient of our local dentist for many years. After I became a chiropractor, I ran into him and we talked about the perils of owning your own practice, all the difficult decisions you have to make and the hats you have to wear. One of the trickiest components of practice ownership is that if you take a week's vacation, your practice loses momentum in your absence. All those new patients you would have seen don't get attended to, and once you return it is exhausting trying to catch up with the patients and the business issues you missed while away. A week or two off becomes a huge stress and perhaps not worth it in the end.

My dentist told me that he discovered a way to have a successful vacation without any of the downsides. He brought up a calendar of the ten weeks in summer. He said, "Now a doctor might take a week off in June and one off in August to spend with family and enjoy the summer. But then many of the weeks of summer are spent preparing to get out of town, or cleaning up the backlog after they get back. To solve for this, I decided to take vertical weeks off." He pointed to the Monday and Tuesday of each week and said, "Through the summer, I take Mondays and Tuesdays as vacation. This means I get twenty days off during the summer with less impact to the practice. I am gone 30 percent of the summer, but my patients don't feel my absence, and the routine is healthier and more sustainable."

When I was designing *The Three Day Reset*, I was reminded of this conversation. There are many excellent nutrition programs on the market. The "thirty day this" and the "twenty-one day that," but what if there were something more sustainable that you could get your head wrapped around? A smaller chunk to bite off with less impact on your social and home life? I did the math. If you do *The Three Day Reset* once a month, you are eating clean 10 percent of the month. Fantastic! What a great way to cleanse and reset your body for three days every month.

But if you choose to increase the frequency of The Reset, your results could be even more remarkable. Twice a month and you are eating clean 20 percent of the time. Jump to a weekly Reset and 40 percent of your month is pure, perfect nutrition. Forty percent!! Excellent nutrition is ultimately about consistency. I have found in my own personal practice that adhering to a less intense plan executed more consistently yields better benefits and a long-term transformation. Get the most from this program. Make *The Three Day Reset* a consistent part of your nutrition practice.

> "Pure, perfect nutrition 40 percent of the time!"

THE EXECUTION

Upon Waking:
One cup of lemon water tea and a probiotic (wait thirty minutes before taking greens).

One Half Hour Later:
One scoop of greens formula in six ounces of cold water.

Mid morning:
Half of your green smoothie (put the other half in the fridge).

Late Morning:
One cup bone broth. Heat as you would tea or a light soup.

Midday:
Two or more cups of salad with a fish or chicken portion. Toss salad with a drizzle of dressing and either heat your chicken or slice it and have it cold on top of the salad.

Mid Afternoon:
Second half of your smoothie.

Late Day:
Two or more cups of vegetables, sauteed or steamed, with a portion of chicken or fish.

Evening:
One cup of bone broth.

Before Bed:
Probiotic

Drink your lemon water tea as soon after waking as possible. Your greens should be one-half hour after that. As for the rest of the meals, listen to your body and eat when you are hungry. If you are hungry between meals, you can have some additional bone broth, veggies, or a one to two ounce serving of fish or chicken. Do not snack on anything else. Drink lots and lots of water. (I prefer half my body weight in ounces.)

Sauté

1. Chop vegetables and meat or fish to a similar size.
2. Heat a small amount of avocado oil in a wok or skillet on medium-high.
3. Add meat or fish and cook for two to four minutes.
4. Add vegetables and cook for another six minutes.
5. Add coconut aminos or a dash of water to provide some moisture.

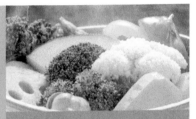

Steaming

1. Chop vegetables to a consistent size. (Denser vegetables should be cut smaller than those vegetables that will cook more quickly.)
2. Add vegetables to a steamer or a pot with a steamer basket with a small amount of water in the bottom.
3. Cover the pot and cook with steam until vegetables are tender.
4. Remove vegetables from heat as soon as they are done, as they will continue to steam and easily overcook.
5. Enjoy with a serving of meat or fish.

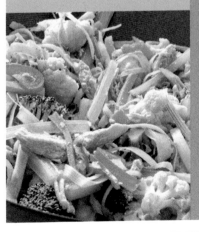

THE BOOSTERS

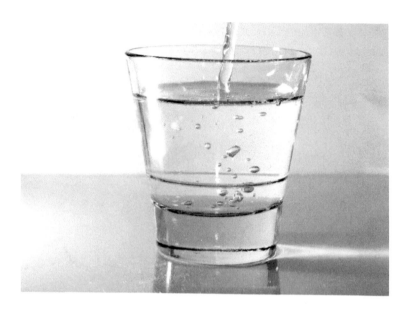

Do you want to get even more out of your *Three Day Reset* process? Add any or all of these boosters for an even more powerful experience.

1. **Hot bath with two to three cups of Epsom salts:** (You can also add essential oils.) Soak for at least twenty minutes and drink lots of water before and after.

2. **Infrared sauna sessions:** Infrared heat is therapeutic and detoxifying. There are many local gyms and yoga studios that have saunas now, so check around.

3. **Extra lemon water tea:** You can have as many cups of this as you like!

4. **More sleep:** If possible, try to go to bed earlier than usual. Remove all distractions and tech from the bedroom while you are "Resetting." If you are able go without an alarm in the morning, that is the best.

5. **Intentional schedule clearing:** Be merciless. Use these three days as a time to rest and simplify. Practice just saying "no!"

6. **Meditation:** Even just deep breathing, observing nature, and napping can be considered forms of meditation. Try to incorporate some intentional miniquiet times during your three days.

7. **Water, water, water!!** At least half your body weight in ounces or three liters, whichever is greater.

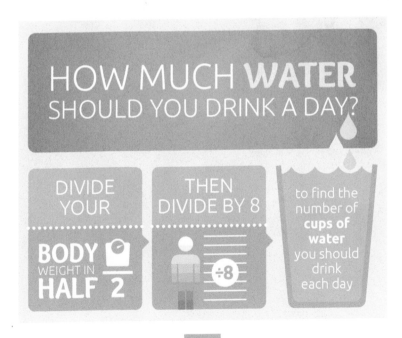

THE SHOP

Put simply, you need ingredients for your smoothies, enough veggies for three salads and three sautés or steamed meals. You need your protein sources, greens, probiotics, lemon for hot lemon water tea, and either homemade or store-bought organic bone broth. I have compiled a sample shopping list below for you to use.

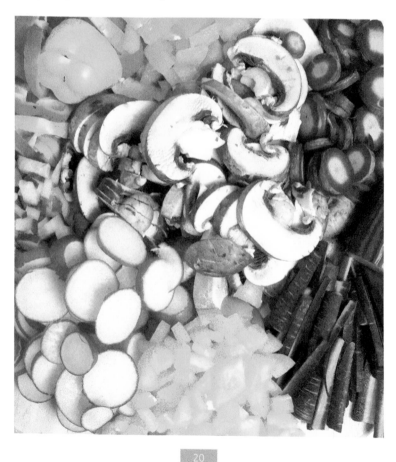

Sample Shopping List

Chicken (antibiotic free, organic) 3 breasts

Salmon (unfarmed) 1.5 lbs (Can also use Halibut)

Avocado oil

Sesame oil

Red wine vinegar

Apple cider vinegar/ White wine vinegar

Garlic powder

Ginger powder

Salt/Pepper

Fresh ginger (At least three good size 1-inch chunks)

Spinach – 10 cups

Kale – If you want to use it for sauté, salads, or smoothies

Bananas – 2 (½ per smoothie)

Organic blueberries (frozen is fine) – 3 cups

Lettuce for three salads

Tomatoes – 2

Cucumbers – 2

Avocados – 2

Green onion – one bunch

Radishes – 1-2 bunches

Stir-fry veggies (example: mushrooms, peppers, zucchini, broccoli, red onion – enough for three steamed or sautéed meals)

Lemon juice – at least one cup to use for smoothies and lemon tea.

Coconut Aminos – I like to add this to anything I sauté for delicious added flavor.

Organic Bone Broth (If you are not making your own)

Online Sources:

Greens Formula: Nanogreens

Protein Powder: Vital Proteins / Pumpkin Protein

Bone Broth: Pacific Natural Organic Broth / US Wellness Meats

Probiotic: Innate Choice / Pure Encapsulations

Fish Oil: Zinzino / Innate Choice

Flavor For Stir-Fry: Coconut Aminos

See references for details.

REMINDERS

1. Remember that all ingredients should be organic and well-sourced.
2. Your purchases online will last you through several Resets.
3. Remember that you can make whatever marinade for the chicken and or fish that you like as long as you don't stray outside the rules of *The Three Day Reset*.
4. Feel free to use any salad dressing that meets *The Three Day Reset* "allowable list."

THE RECIPES

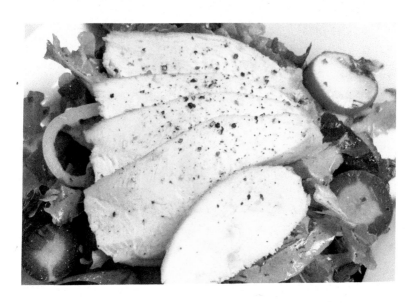

Red Wine Vinegar Chicken

INGREDIENTS

3 Boneless breasts of chicken

¼ cup avocado oil (can substitute olive oil)

⅓ cup red wine vinegar

1 tsp. garlic powder

1 tsp. ginger powder

¼ tsp. sesame oil

Salt – dash

Pepper – dash

Cayenne pepper – optional (¼ tsp.)

INSTRUCTIONS

1. Preheat oven to 350 degrees Fahrenheit.
2. Rinse chicken breasts and pat dry.
3. Gently cut three slices into each breast, ¼ inch deep on the bias or grain of the meat. (Optional – Improves marinade process).
4. Combine marinade ingredients together in a jar or shaker and mix well.
5. Place breasts of chicken into a mixing bowl and pour marinade over top.
6. Mix chicken with marinade and let sit for 15 minutes.
7. Line a cookie sheet with foil and place breasts on foil
8. Place chicken into a preheated oven for 20-25 minutes or until an internal temperature of 165 degrees Fahrenheit is achieved. (See note about pan searing below.)
9. Let chicken cool and serve warm or cold with vegetables or salad.

A NOTE ON PAN SEARING

I actually like to "pan sear" breasts of chicken that I am baking. Pan searing gives the chicken a prettier finished look and it seals in moisture and reduces baking time. To pan sear, heat a frying pan on the stove with coconut or avocado oil (1-2 Tbsp.). Let the pan get nice and warm. Gently place the chicken in the pan and let sear for 1-2 minutes per side, and then place chicken on baking pan and into the oven and bake as directed.

Three Day Reset Smoothie

INGREDIENTS

2 cups or large handfuls of spinach

½ banana ≈ 10 slices

½ cup of blueberries

¼ avocado

⅓ cucumber ≈ 10 slices

½ cup ice

1-2 scoops of allowable protein powder (see recommendations)

½ lemon, juiced

1-2 inches fresh ginger (I just wash the outside and throw it in; no need to peel!)

⅛ - ¼ cup of water – You can always add more if your smoothie is too thick.

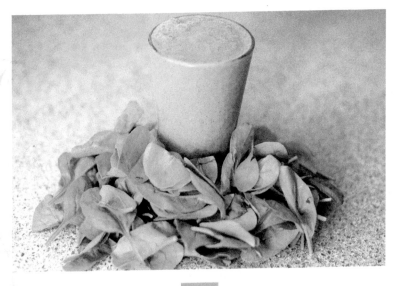

INSTRUCTIONS

1. Add all ingredients to a blender.
2. Blend really well!
3. Split contents into two containers.
4. Drink one! Save the second for later.

OPTIONAL BOOSTS FOR YOUR SMOOTHIE:

If you want to supercharge this smoothie you can add any or all of the following: a good pharmaceutical grade fish oil, liquid vitamin D, glutamine, or hemp seeds for some added protein and fiber. *(see resources)*

Lemon Water Tea

1. Heat a cup of water to boiling.
2. Add the juice of half a lemon.
3. Drink and enjoy!

Basic Salad Dressing

INGREDIENTS

¼ cup avocado oil
¼ cup white wine vinegar or apple cider vinegar
¼ lemon, juiced
Pinch of salt and pepper
One clove garlic, minced
Spices of your choice – oregano, rosemary, basil

INSTRUCTIONS

Mix all ingredients well in an enclosed container. Keeps in the fridge for up to two weeks.

Bone Broth Recipe

For the purposes of *The Three Day Reset*, we are going to be using chicken bone broth. If you elect to purchase your bone broth, here are three trusted resources. Be sure to purchase organic, and, if in the future you are using beef broth, be sure to get grass-fed organic.

- **Thrive Market:** https://thrivemarket.com/
- **Vitacost:** http://www.vitacost.com/
- **Amazon:** https://www.amazon.com/

If you choose to make your own, it is easy and significantly cheaper!

INGREDIENTS

2 pounds of chicken bones – About two to three deboned chickens per gallon of soup is a good rule to stick to.

¼ cup of apple cider vinegar

Filtered water to cover bones

2 carrots, chopped

2 stalks of celery, chopped

1 onion, chopped

OPTIONAL:

You can add parsley, salt, pepper, other spices like oregano and rosemary, and you can add cloves of garlic for the last 30 minutes of cooking.

INSTRUCTIONS

1. Acquire your bones! Here's how:
   a. Roast an organic chicken or two, eat, and then voila! You have bones to use.
   b. Contact your local butcher for pastured, organic, chicken bones.
   c. Contact your local farmer.
   d. Contact US Wellness Meats: http://grasslandbeef.com/ PH: (877) 383-0051
2. Add bones to a large stockpot on the stove. (If you are using raw bones, first roast them in the oven at 350 degrees Fahrenheit until brown and then transfer to your broth pot.)
3. Add water so that the level is 1.5 to 2 inches above the bones. You can always add water as time passes if the broth appears to be getting too thick.
4. Add ¼ cup of apple cider vinegar.
5. Let sit in cold water for 30 minutes. Cold water will better allow the flavor to be brought out of the bones.
6. Add carrots, celery, onion, and any of the optional ingredients to the pot and turn the stove to high.
7. Bring to a boil for two minutes and then turn down to low and cover.
8. It is good to check on the stock every 20 minutes for the first 4 hours and remove any impurities floating on the top with a large spoon.
9. Cover and let cook on low heat for a total 8-24 hours. The longer bone broth cooks, the better!
10. Once finished, strain soup through cheesecloth or a metal strainer to catch the bones and vegetables.
    You might see some gelatin form as the soup is cooling. This is GOOD!! This is liquid gold. Do not get rid of it!
11. Place in mason jars in the fridge or freezer until ready for use.

Thank you to Wellness Mama, Kellyann Petrucci, and Laura Foster DC for inspiring this bone broth recipe.

BONE BROTH BASICS

Yes, I know. Drinking the broth of bones may not be what you had in mind when you started considering *The Three Day Reset*. I have had participants ask if they could omit this portion of the program, and my firm, unwavering response is "No!" Here's why:

Let us first discuss how bone broth is different than chicken or beef stock. Bone broth is loaded with rich quantities of collagen, proteins, and minerals traditionally absent in regular stock or broths. You will also notice a slightly thicker texture to bone broth. This is due to the collagen that is released from the bones during cooking. The taste is also richer. The reason why bone broth can be considered a secret weapon of *The Three Day Reset* is due to the multitude of benefits it provides. The following list shares many of the attributes of bone broth:

Digestion: Both the amino acids glycine and glutamine are essential for proper functioning of the gut, and in conditions like Irritable Bowel Syndrome or Leaky Gut, their absence can be devastating. Bone broth provides copious amounts of both these essential nutrients.

Joint Health: During the cooking process, bones and tendons are broken down into gelatin. Gelatin, the part that creates the thickness in broth, is rich in the amino acids proline and glycine. These two bad boys are the building blocks for connective tissue like muscles, ligaments, and tendons. Achy or arthritic joints often experience relief with supplementation of gelatin or gelatin-containing foods like bone broth.

Anti-Inflammatory: Bone broth contains glucosamine and chondroitin sulfate. You have probably heard these names because of supplements containing these nutrients. These supplements have become popular because of their influence over inflammation. Well, in bone broth, you can get both glucosamine and chondroitin right from your cup. These two natural constituents of cartilage are believed to act as soothing joint anti-inflammatories. They are also thought to assist in cartilage repair.

Detoxification: The high amounts of glycine in bone broth accomplish at least three essential functions related to the detoxification process. Glycine aids the liver in removing toxins. It is also an essential part of glutathione synthesis. (Glutathione is one of the most important antioxidants in our body.) It also helps clear away methionine. Methionine is an essential amino acid, but too much of it in the system can lead to trouble.

Minerals: Bone broth is rich in the minerals calcium, potassium, magnesium, and phosphorous. These four minerals are often deficient in our bodies, particularly for women. Bone broth is an excellent way to deliver highly absorbable nutrients to keep your mineral balances optimal. It is impossible to determine the exact mineral amount present if you make broth at home because you can't know how much is released from the bones, but any additional mineral support we can get is going to aid generalized healing, cardiac function, and immune resilience.

Marrow: Predatory animals have it down. They will scoop up bones of their kill and smash them on rocks or crack them open with their teeth so they can drink the marrow inside. Besides being delicious, marrow is rich with building blocks for many systems of our body, including bone growth and development. The high marrow content in bone broth means you are drinking healthy fats, essential minerals, and key building blocks with every steaming mug.

Now you know why this nutrient-dense golden liquid is an essential part of *The Three Day Reset* plan. Whether you make your bone broth at home or purchase it from one of the online resources provided, your two cups a day are an intentional component of rebuilding and revitalizing your health.

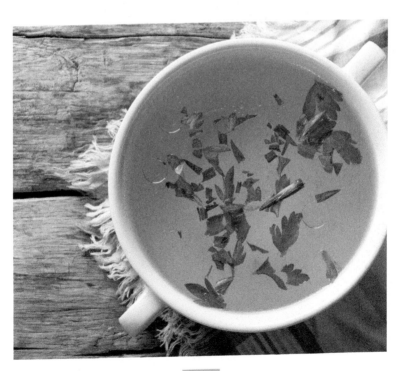

THE POWER PREP

You can use the recipes I have provided for you, or you can use your own recipes as long as you follow the guidelines of the "not allowed" list. Please note that you can sauté, steam, bake, or roast your food. You may also choose to grill your meat – just be sure to avoid charring.

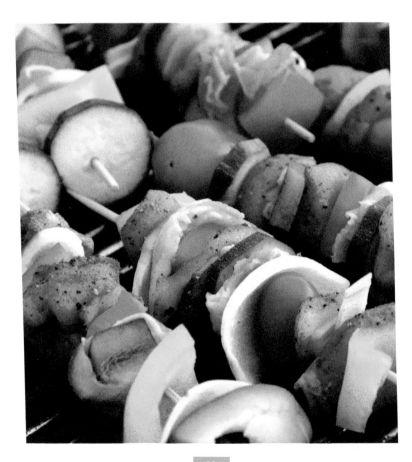

Power Prep Instructions

- Turn oven onto 375 degrees Fahrenheit.

- When the oven is ready, brush salmon with avocado oil, salt, and pepper, and bake for 15 minutes or until the internal temperature reads 125 degrees Fahrenheit.

- While fish is cooking, make the chicken marinade (see recipe below) and allow the chicken to marinate for 15 minutes.

- Take out salmon when it reaches its appropriate internal temperature of 125 degrees Fahrenheit and put the chicken in at the same temperature of 375 degrees Fahrenheit. Cook chicken for approximately 20-22 minutes or until internal temperature is 165 degrees Fahrenheit.

- While chicken is cooking and salmon is cooling, make enough salad dressing for at least three salads and put in the fridge. (Alternatively, you can just drizzle olive/avocado oil and vinegar on your salads with a little dash of salt and pepper.)

- When the chicken reaches its appropriate internal temperature, take it out and let cool.

- Now wash all of your vegetables including lettuce, spinach, and kale. (If using kale, cut it into bite-size pieces after washing.)

- Place clean, dried, prepped lettuces (spinach, salad lettuce, kale) in large freezer bags or glass containers with either a dishtowel or paper towel to soak up any excess moisture. Place in the refrigerator.

- Portion salmon into thirds and place in glass containers.

- Place cooled chicken breasts in glass containers and place in the refrigerator.

- Start chopping vegetables into appropriate sizes for sautés/steaming/salads. Separate out your portions for each meal, seal in a glass container, and place in the refrigerator.

- Clean up!

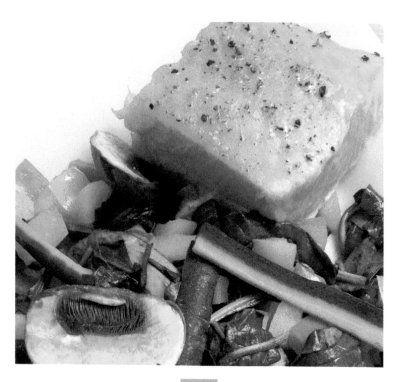

THE FAQS

1. **Will I lose weight on *The Three Day Reset*?** Likely, but it depends on your body composition and typical eating habits. It is probable that your bowels are going to start mobilizing more efficiently, and candidly, you are just going to have less junk stuck in the pipes. That may account for some initial weight loss. You may also lose some water as your body starts to adjust to clean eating. However, if you practice *The Three Day Reset* regularly, you will lose weight IF your body needs to lose weight.

2. **Is *The Three Day Reset* safe?** YES! Not just safe, but frankly, for some it is a life preserver to a drowning man. We often don't realize the level of nutrient body abuse to which we have slowly grown accustomed. *The Three Day Reset* eliminates the unsafe practices in our diets, such as the consumption of toxins, processed foods, chemicals, and allergens.

3. **Why am I giving up red meat and pork?** There is absolutely nothing wrong with red meat and pork if it is WELL-SOURCED. The problem is that red meat and pork are proteins for which it is most difficult to ensure good farming practices. (Chicken can also be risky business unless you are sure you are getting organic, antibiotic-free birds, so if you are not confident of your meat quality, stick with fresh, un-farmed, well-sourced fish.)

4. **Why only salmon or halibut?** Unfortunately, our general fish population is laden with heavy metals. In my opinion, there are many fish out there you shouldn't consume, like salmon and roughy. Again, the cleanest, most readily available fishes are salmon and halibut.

5. **Why is there so little fruit and no fruit juice?** Fruits are excellent sources of vitamins and other nutrients, but your body also sees them as sugar underneath all that lovely color and texture. One half of a banana in your smoothie and one cup of frozen blueberries are all that is allowed per day.

6. **Why am I giving up all grains, dairy, and eggs?** These foods provoke the most common food sensitivities. Even if a food sensitivity test says you are clear of any sensitivities, it is tricky to know for sure if you are internally reacting to these aggravators. It is best to occasionally eliminate them to give your tract a little break.

7. **Can I do *The Three Day Reset* for more than three days at a time?** Yes! There is nothing about *The Three Day Reset* that is unsafe for longer periods of time. But three days is enough time to give your body a rest and derive significant benefit. The Reset is also a good launch point for those new to dietary adjustments and whole food eating.

8. **How often do you commit to *The Three Day Reset?*** I have been practicing *The Three Day Reset* for some time now to refine and perfect it for you! I have found that doing *The Three Day Reset* Monday, Tuesday, and Wednesday of every week is a manageable practice that has yielded exceptional results over time. But once a month is the minimum recommended frequency.

9. **What if I don't have time to make my bone broth?** See the references to find reputable places to purchase organic, well-sourced bone broth.

10. **Why do I feel like crap the first time I do *The Three Day Reset?*** Ahhhh, yes, very common reaction. When your body is sensitive to certain things, it is not very happy at first after you take that "inflammation feeder" away. Also, yeast overgrowth in your intestinal tract gets very upset (flu-like symptoms) once it stops being fed sugar! Stick it out, rest more, try to do baths or saunas, and drink copious amounts of water. Trust me, as you keep implementing the reset, this reaction will improve. Think of it as your body going through deep healing.

11. **I am paleo or gluten and dairy free. Why would I need *The Three Day Reset?*** Good for you! *The Three Day Reset* will be easy for you. Eliminating natural sweeteners, red meat, and pork will be a nice additional break for your body. Frankly, I find most of my clients practice the "80/20 rule" of paleo, so going 100 percent paleo a few days a month or a few days a week is a fantastic additional choice for your body.

12. **What are some other things I can do to boost *The Three Day Reset?*** Infrared sauna, hot epsom salt baths with lavender or other detoxifying oils, additional lemon water tea, more sleep, meditation, and intentional schedule clearing will help you get the most out of *The Three Day Reset*.

13. **What if I feel no differently on *The Three Day Reset?*** You will, but if you don't, remember that marvelous things are occurring under the surface. The operations of purging toxins, decreasing inflammation, and populating good gut bacteria may not have demonstrative signs at first, but over time you will begin to see changes.

14. **Am I actually "detoxifying" my liver?** In my opinion, no. Your liver is perfectly capable of detoxifying itself. That is the liver's job. HOWEVER, when you bombard an organ with too many tasks all at once (like eating crap for dozens of years), it may not perform as effectively as it could. *The Three Day Reset* gives your liver a wee rest from such intense demand.

15. **Can I work out while I am on *The Three Day Reset?*** Yes, and feel free to increase your protein portions if your workout demands are high.

16. **What if I am hungry on *The Three Day Reset?*** Often, "hunger signals" can be boredom or anxiousness. Recognize the hunger pangs for what they are. Try to stick to the recommendations. (Part of giving our bodies a break is eating less for the three days. You will not die of hunger in three days!) BUT, if you need to add more food, start with more vegetables and bone broth and then protein, if necessary.

17. **I will die without coffee!** Then have it, but get well-sourced, good quality coffee and have it black. One to two cups only, please.

18. **I am a vegetarian. Can I still do *the Three Day Reset*?** The reset is geared toward meat eaters. Because of the elimination of legumes and grains, it would be difficult for a vegetarian to get the proper protein needed for a healthy execution of *The Three Day Reset*.

19. **Can I use any greens powder, or does it have to be Nanogreens?** In the twenty years I have been practicing and coaching clients on nutrition, I have not found a better, more absorbable greens powder. If you find one that you love, and it has excellent ingredients and sourcing, then of course, use it. I promote Nanogreens because the taste is the best on the market, the producer sources the ingredients of Nanogreens with excellent intention, and it has Phytosorb, which helps the nutritious ingredients get past the gut wall. (See references for purchasing information.)

20. **Should I be taking my other supplements while on *The Three Day Reset*?** For the most part, the answer is no. It is okay to take a break for a few days, with the exception of your probiotic, greens, and a recommended fish oil. Many readily available supplements have binders, contaminants, and processing practices that can contribute to leaky gut and dietary issues. Many have soy and dairy in them. Best to just take a break for the three days and then reintroduce them after if need be. **If you are under the guidance of a doctor or naturopath, seek his or her counsel before making decisions to halt the use of supplements or medications.**

DAILY JOURNAL

Do you use food as something other than fuel? Is food your friend? Is food a way to fill the void, cure boredom, or make you forget? Behaviors and emotions toward food are deeply rooted from the time we are very young. As you generate consciousness around your eating over these three days, it will set the stage for personal reflection on how food affects you.

The opportunity to journal during this program can provide a deepening of your transformation. Journaling is a chance to spill onto paper your thoughts, feelings, and realizations around your relationships with trigger foods. Where are your cravings the strongest? What conversation goes on in your head as you negotiate between sticking with the program or not?

Can you get excellent benefit from the *The Three Day Reset* without journaling? Yes! Your body is still going to feel alive and you will feel more energized and alert. However, if you want to reap even more of the benefits, allotting time for journaling can be a key element of success.

Here are some prompt questions to get you going.

JOURNAL QUESTIONS

1. What am I grateful for?
2. What elements of my health feel good right now?
3. What elements of my health would I like to improve?
4. What cravings am I experiencing?
5. What emotions am I having in direct relationship to the foods that are on the "not allowed list"?
6. Do I ever experience negative emotions like anger or self-hatred around the food choices I have made? From where does that stem?
7. What has most surprised me in this program so far?
8. Is there anything that hurts today?
9. Am I feeling "detoxy" at all?
10. What are the reasons I am doing *The Three Day Reset*?
11. What have I learned about myself so far in the program?
12. What new behaviors would I like to continue after the three days are up?
13. How can I be kinder to myself today?

All of these observations can help transform your relationship with food. Taking just a few minutes every day to journal is an essential part of the process. I have included enough pages here for four *Three Day Resets*. You can get additional copies on WELLFITandFED anytime.

If you have food behaviors such as binging, purging, or withholding, reach out to a local food behavior professional for help.

THE THREE DAY RESET JOURNAL

Day 1   **Day 2**   **Day 3**

Gratitude:

Thoughts and Impressions:

Action Steps and Affirmations:

THE THREE DAY RESET JOURNAL

Day 1   **Day 2**   **Day 3**

Gratitude:

Thoughts and Impressions:

Action Steps and Affirmations:

THE THREE DAY RESET JOURNAL

Day 1   **Day 2**   **Day 3**

Gratitude:

Thoughts and Impressions:

Action Steps and Affirmations:

THE THREE DAY RESET JOURNAL

Day 1   **Day 2**   **Day 3**

Gratitude:

Thoughts and Impressions:

Action Steps and Affirmations:

THE THREE DAY RESET JOURNAL

Day 1   **Day 2**   **Day 3**

Gratitude:

Thoughts and Impressions:

Action Steps and Affirmations:

THE THREE DAY RESET JOURNAL

Day 1   **Day 2**   **Day 3**

Gratitude:

Thoughts and Impressions:

Action Steps and Affirmations:

THE THREE DAY RESET JOURNAL

Day 1　　　　　　**Day 2**　　　　　　**Day 3**

Gratitude:

Thoughts and Impressions:

Action Steps and Affirmations:

THE THREE DAY RESET JOURNAL

Day 1   **Day 2**   **Day 3**

Gratitude:

Thoughts and Impressions:

Action Steps and Affirmations:

THE THREE DAY RESET JOURNAL

Day 1   **Day 2**   **Day 3**

Gratitude:

Thoughts and Impressions:

Action Steps and Affirmations:

THE THREE DAY RESET JOURNAL

Day 1   **Day 2**   **Day 3**

Gratitude:

Thoughts and Impressions:

Action Steps and Affirmations:

THE THREE DAY RESET JOURNAL

Day 1   **Day 2**   **Day 3**

Gratitude:

Thoughts and Impressions:

Action Steps and Affirmations:

THE THREE DAY RESET JOURNAL

Day 1   **Day 2**   **Day 3**

Gratitude:

Thoughts and Impressions:

Action Steps and Affirmations:

LIFE AFTER RESET

So you have completed *The Three Day Reset* one or more times, and you are wondering how to nutritionally behave for the rest of the week. That is a great question! The beauty of *The Three Day Reset* is that it provides flexibility in your week, so you don't have to be militant in your approach to food. If you do *The Three Day Reset* as recommended, it translates to perfect nutrition for 40 percent of your month. Not many people can say they eat perfectly 40 percent of the time! During the Reset days, you are filling your body with well-sourced healthy meats, fresh organic fruits and vegetables, nutrient-dense bone broth, and an antioxidant-packed anti-inflammatory smoothie. What a great investment in your health!

But the question is: What should I do the rest of the time? The first thing to remember is that you can continue portions of the Reset program throughout the rest of your week. There are no adverse effects to an ongoing Reset. If you enjoy the bone broth, then consider continuing with that regimen; if you love the smoothie, make it part of every day. You get the idea. The intent behind *The Three Day Reset* is to bring you back to clean, whole food nutrition and also to establish habits of excellent eating that spill over to the rest of your week.

Food Sensitivities

Another benefit of *The Three Day Reset* is that the plan removes most potential allergens from your diet for three days. This means that once you start reintroducing foods like wheat and dairy after completing the program, you may notice some responses from your body. Your body is an incredible healing machine. Even after eliminating common allergens for just three days, your body can recover enough that, if it is exposed again, it may react strongly to an offensive invader. Pay attention to these responses. Reactions such as gut discomfort (gas and bloating are not normal!), headaches, fatigue, and irritability can be food-related and symptomatic of a food sensitivity. You might consider eliminating that food for good.

Happy Animals

Now that you have learned about well-sourced chicken and cleanly caught unfarmed fish, watch for sourcing as you reintroduce beef and pork. Look for organic, grass-fed meat wherever possible. Shopping "happy animal products" ensures that you are getting the proper balance of omega 3, 6, and 9 fats. Good sourcing also confirms you are not ingesting any hidden antibiotics, hormones, or other nasties in your piece of meat.

Read Labels

During The Reset, you had to read labels to ensure there was no soy, preservatives, or additives in the food you were purchasing for the program. Make it a habit to continue to read ingredients. Remember that artificial sweeteners, soy, colors, additives, and chemicals you can't pronounce are better left outside your body.

The Dirty Fifteen

Fruits and vegetables are better tolerated if you continue to source organic, but if you would prefer to buy non-organic because of cost, steer clear of the dirty fifteen. You should never compromise choosing organic on the following list:

- apples
- peaches
- strawberries
- nectarines
- grapes
- celery
- spinach
- sweet bell peppers
- cucumbers
- cherry tomatoes
- snap peas
- potatoes
- hot peppers
- kale
- collard greens

Source for the The Dirty Dozen Plus: http://www.drweil.com/drw/u/ART02985/Foods-You-Should-Always-Buy-Organic.html

Hello Sweetness

Sweeteners are the most difficult "food" for many to give up. When coming off *The Three Day Reset*, you might consider adding back only natural sugars like stevia, maple syrup, and honey. Avoid refined sweeteners like brown rice syrup, wheat syrup, and high fructose corn syrup. There are so many delicious recipes that utilize only natural sugars. Sugar and artificial sweeteners may not be as difficult to give up as you first thought once you consider the devastating effects that sugar has on alkalinity in the digestive system, gut permeability, and generalized inflammation in the body.

Processed Foods

Think of processed food as anything in a box or a can. Think of processed food as anything with multiple ingredients and a long shelf life. Think of processed food as anything with a commercial. One of the most important choices to entertain as you disembark from *The Three Day Reset* is continuing to avoid processed foods. The impact of preservatives, artificial colors, sweeteners, and questionable chemicals spells disaster for your health.

The Three Day Reset is intended to allow you to eat less strictly for four days of the week. The program is intended to be completely doable by having flexibility. But ask yourself a question: Do your "normal eating habits" need refining? Can you use your time on *The Three Day Reset* as a springboard to make excellent nutritional changes on non-Reset days? Eating well takes practice and discipline. The methods in *The Three Day Reset* will teach you how to make better, more nutritionally conscious choices during the rest of your week.

THE FINAL WORD

If you are reading this book, then I'd better take a moment to commend you. By holding it, reading it, and digesting the information, you communicate to me that you are growing and learning in your pursuit of greater health. I am already proud of you.

Implement *The Three Day Reset* with the long term in mind. You will get excellent benefit from going through the program once, but imagine your results if you set up a once or twice monthly practice. Imagine if you jumped on board weekly! Each time you incorporate a Reset into your week, you will be investing in the "defining and refining" of your practice of exceptional nutrition.

There will be questions as you go. Keep the book handy and return to it as you learn more about the three-day process of eating whole, organic, well-sourced foods. Continue to revisit the journaling section and see what new insights you have about your practice of eating.

Remember that excellent nutrition is a discipline. Like anything we hope to master, we need to keep getting up, dusting off, and starting again when we make choices out of line with our intentions. But each time we take steps forward, we grow stronger, more knowledgeable, and we arm ourselves with great opportunity for success. So as you are embarking on *The Three Day Reset*, be gentle with yourself. This is about progress, not perfection.

As you journey through your three days, I would love to hear from you. I would also be so pleased if you would share this program with others. The more people we can encourage to invest in consistent, clean nutrition, the better everything in our lives will be. Healthy food, healthy bodies, bright minds, tremendous life experiences!

Most of all, I want you to know how grateful I am for you. I believe that you have the ability to live life with the explosive energy and vibrancy that only exceptional nutrition brings.

Now let's Reset!
Heather Denniston DC CCWP

ONLINE RESOURCES

Probiotic for morning and evening:
(Your probiotic should be high quality and should not be shelf-stable. In other words, it should have to be refrigerated.)

Innate Choice
http://www.innatechoice.com/probioticsufficiency.cfm

Pure Encapsulations
http://www.pureencapsulations.com/products/shop-by-product-category/probiotics-prebiotics/probiotic-50b.html

For your greens formula for first thing in the morning:

Nanogreens
http://www.biopharmasci.com/nanogreens-vegetable-supplements-p/1ng10-btl-s.htm

Fish oil for your morning smoothie:

Innate Choice
http://www.innatechoice.com/omegasufficiency.cfm

Zinzino
http://www.izinzino.com/

ONLINE RESOURCES

Vitamin D source booster for your smoothie:

Innate Choice Vitamin D Sufficiency
http://www.innatechoice.com/dsufficiency.cfm

Protein Powder Options:

Vital Proteins:
http://www.vitalproteins.com/collagen/
collagen-peptides.html

Pumpkin Protein Powder
https://www.amazon.com/Omega-Nutrition-Pumpkin-
Protein-21-Ounce/dp/
B004L3VLFK?ie=UTF8&*Version*=1&*entries*=0

Glutamine – excellent for digestion during
The Three Day Reset:
http://www.pureencapsulations.com/

Coconut Aminos that you can add to stir-frys:

http://www.vitacost.com/coconut-secret-the-original-
coconut-aminos-soy-free-seasoning-sauce

ONLINE RESOURCES

All-purpose herbs for salads and stir-frys:

Simply Organic All Purpose Seasoning
http://www.vitacost.com/simply-organic-all-purpose-
seasoning

Organic bone broth options:

Thrive Market
https://thrivemarket.com/

Vitacost
http://www.vitacost.com/

Amazon
https://www.amazon.com/

Grass Fed Meats:

US Wellness Meats
http://grasslandbeef.com/

Epsom salts for your Epsom salt baths:

Dr. Teals
https://www.amazon.com/Dr-Teals-Lavender-Epsom-Salt/
dp/B003GC4GH2?ie=UTF8&*Version*=1&*entries*=0

LINKS & INFLUENCERS

BOOKS

Dr. Kellyann's Bone Broth Diet - Kellyann Petrucci, ND

Your Body's Many Cries For Water - F. Batmanghelidj, MD

It Starts With Food - Dallas and Melissa Hartwig

Lick The Sugar Habit - Nancy Appleton

The Sugar Blues - William Duffy

Eat Fat, Get Thin - Mark Hyman, MD

Brain Rules - John Medina

The Wellness Prevention Paradigm
- James Chestnut, DC CCWP

Brain Maker by David Perlmutter, MD

The Primal Blueprint - Mark Sisson

Breaking the Habit of Being Yourself - Joe Dispenza, DC

Daring Greatly - Brené Brown

Wheat Belly - William Davis, MD

LINKS & INFLUENCERS

FILMS

That Sugar Film

Fat Sick & Nearly Dead

Fast Food Nation

WEBSITES

Against All Grain

Civilized Caveman

PaleoLeap

PaleoOMG

Organic Kitchen

Deliciously Ella

Oh She Glows

The Sprouted Kitchen

Lexi's Clean Kitchen

Nom Nom Paleo

Author Bio

Heather Denniston is a seasoned chiropractor with advanced certifications in pediatrics, pregnancy, and Wellness Chiropractic (CCWP). She is an avid athlete, optimal health enthusiast, and writer who has a passion for inspiring people of all ages to ignite first steps toward realizing their greatness within. Through online content, public speaking, and coaching, Heather shares wellness, fitness, and nutrition expertise for those looking for deeper change. Dr. Denniston splits her time between Issaquah, Washington and Scottsdale, Arizona. If you are interested in a consultation, or in hiring her as a speaker or writer, she can always be found at her blog, WELLFITandFED.com.